THE RECOVERY LIFESTYLE

THE RECOVERY LIFESTYLE

How to Leave Addiction Behind, Get Excited About
Life, and Become the Person You Deserve to Be

ANDRÉ VIEL

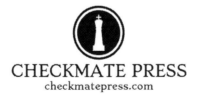

CHECKMATE PRESS

checkmatepress.com

Checkmate Press books are published by:

McLean Media Group, LLC
4364 Glenwood Dr
Bozeman, Montana 59718 USA
www.checkmatepress.com
www.mcleanmedia.com

The Recovery Lifestyle / André Viel. -- 1st ed.
ISBN 978-1-7321781-2-0

The Publisher has strived to be as accurate and complete as possible in the creation of this book.

This book is not intended for use as a source of legal, business, accounting, or financial advice. All readers are advised to seek services of competent professionals in legal, business, accounting, and finance field.

In practical advice books, like anything else in life, there are no guarantees of income or results made. Readers are cautioned to rely on their own judgment about their individual circumstances to act accordingly.

While all attempts have been made to verify information provided in this publication, the Publisher assumes no responsibility for errors, omissions, or contrary interpretation of the subject matter herein. Any perceived slights of specific persons, peoples, or organizations are unintentional.

This book is not intended as a substitute for the medical advice of physicians. The reader should regularly consult a physician in matters relating to his/her health and particularly with respect to any symptoms that may require diagnosis or medical attention.

This book is dedicated to all those still suffering in silence, may you find the spark that ignites your hope and leads you to a path of recovery and healing.

I'd also like to dedicate this book to my son, he's been my hope, my inspiration, and his unconditional love is a big reason I'm alive today to write this book. Love you Maxim.

TABLE OF CONTENTS

PART ONE:

INTRODUCTION

CHAPTER 1:
WHY ADOPT A RECOVERY LIFESTYLE?

Focus on building a recovery lifestyle, and your goals will follow.

The Recovery Lifestyle includes making choices that are conducive to your health and your recovery, and that aligns with your values and life goals. Recovery lifestyle is different for everyone but can be one of the biggest tools and life-changing decisions helping you on your path to healing from addiction, depression, or many other challenges.

Have you ever heard people trying to lose weight say, "It's not a diet, it's a lifestyle?" Well, it turns out that there is a lot of truth to this. Have you ever noticed (or maybe experienced for yourself) how people go on and off diets their whole life, but never really see much progress? But when someone starts the journey toward a healthy lifestyle, they often can achieve amazing lifelong results. They improve their health, increased energy, and lose weight, but those are all byproducts of focusing energy on a healthy lifestyle instead of losing weight.

Same goes with addiction recovery.

If you chase and focus all your energy on sobriety or a specific harm reduction goal, you're essentially putting energy into a diet. Instead, create a Recovery Lifestyle that works for you.

There are guidelines for creating a healthy balanced recovery lifestyle, but recovery is personal and can look and be defined differently by different people. And that's ok. That's what's nice about planning out your Recovery Lifestyle. You set it up to be in line with your recovery goals, capabilities, and timeline.

In this book, I will talk about addiction, some information for families of a loved one going through addiction and a step by step guide on how to create a healthy Recovery Lifestyle.

If you are a loved one reading this book to support someone through addiction, then the best first step you can take is to adopt a Recovery Lifestyle yourself. Addiction takes its toll on everyone, not just the person in active addiction. The best way to support recovery is to model it for the person you are trying to support.

The first step to doing this is to take some time and respond to the questions on the following pages.

If you are someone reading this who is in active addiction, then take some time and respond to the questions for yourself.

Either way, it is important to take the time to think about the answers. If you are unsure, it's ok to research to understand better.

~

How would you rate your contentment with the following areas of your life?

1=very discontent, 3=neutral, 5=incredibly satisfied

Career/ Professional Life

1   2   3   4   5

Relationships

1   2   3   4   5

Finances

1   2   3   4   5

Nutrition

1   2   3   4   5

Fitness

1   2   3   4   5

Self-Care

1   2   3   4   5

Sleeping Habits

1   2   3   4   5

Continual Learning

1   2   3   4   5

What are your biggest goals for recovery?

What do you currently do to support recovery?

What are the top things you think you could do to strengthen recovery?

CHAPTER 2:
ANDRE'S STORY

Why am I so passionate about addiction recovery?

"SOMETIMES IT TAKES MORE COURAGE TO ASK FOR HELP THAN TO ACT ALONE "
- KEN PETTI

I'm André Viel, born and raised in a very small town called St- Francois in New Brunswick, Canada. As a child, I had numerous operations on my eardrums (five operations before the age of ten) and needed to learn to cope with the regular fear of surgery and with hearing loss.

I am the middle child of three kids, and my father is one of the managers of the major employer that employs most of the community. Being the boy of a man that is most people's boss brought on a lot of pressure for me as a child. I grew up with the perception I had to be perfect to be loved or accepted by the community and my family. Emotions, especially sad ones, were not understood and not well accepted by my father. My mother was also battling health issues and was not emotionally available at the time.

So, I learned to put on a mask, and I learned that hiding my emotions was the way to please my society and my family. This defense mechanism served me well when I was young, but as an adult, it became more and more of a burden.

I spent so much time putting masks on and focusing my attention on pleasing others that unknowingly I had never gotten to know my true self. I had no real identity and felt a void inside.

But overall, life was manageable until my separation with my high school sweetheart of twelve years, the mother of my son. After that separation, life became more and more unbearable. I was going through verbal and mental abuse in the workplace and experienced a burnout so intense I had to leave my job.

Then I began to believe that I needed a partner to be able to cope with life. And because of my dysfunctional mindset, I ended up in a very toxic relationship. This partner, impacted by mental health challenges, became very manipulative and verbally, mentally, and physically abusive. Nonetheless, I stayed in this relationship for three years trying to heal from my burn out.

In those three years, I was miss-diagnosed by my family doctor with bipolar type two. I was taken off depression meds and put on a very strong mood stabilizer and other medications. Since I was misdiagnosed, these medications made me feel crazy and out of control. I didn't know if I was happy or sad or angry and felt very emotionally unstable.

After an eight-month wait to see a psychiatrist, the psychiatrist confirmed that I was not bipolar. After further testing, I was diagnosed with severe ADHD, anxiety, and depression.

I stopped taking the bipolar medication, and my life started getting better. I got out of the toxic relationship and got into a healthier one. I started a cleaning and painting business, and all in all, things were going well.

But one night, I was out for my birthday and got unfairly targeted and then jumped by a gang of five large men. They beat me, kicked me, and bounced my head on the pavement like a basketball. The bruises, cuts, and physical pain healed, but the emotional pain tormented me and turned into PTSD. I slowly pushed all my friends away and instead turned towards the drug world and gangs.

Anxiety and panic attacks started, and depression hit me like a ton of bricks. I couldn't get out of bed to run my business anymore. I didn't trust the medical system because of past mistakes, so I decided to self-medicate with a speed pill (amphetamine) in the morning. Boom, it worked, and I was able to get out of bed. But snorting one a day became two, then three and only increased. I had smoked marijuana every day since I was eighteen, but had rules around my use and used it more recreationally and to help with sleep or focus for my ADHD. But once I started using speed, my marijuana consumption went up with my speed consumption, and in the end, I was using between ten to fifteen speed pills per day, one ounce of marijuana per week, and high amounts of cocaine and MDMA on the weekend.

I became delusional with suicidal thoughts. My girlfriend had left me a few months prior, and I was convinced that she had hacked into my phone and computer and knew about my drug use, and the kind of people with whom I had been hanging out. I was certain that's why she left me and became obsessed with talking to her to try to explain everything. I kept emailing, messaging and calling and ended up making her and her families Christmas hell, all because I was high and delusional. I ended up scaring this ex-girlfriend and her sister to the point that they filed criminal charges of harassment against me. On one day on the phone with her, her pleas for me to stop finally sunk in. Hearing the anger and fear in her voice had a big impact on me.

The next day, in a moment of sobriety, I called my parents, allowed myself to be vulnerable, and opened up to them about my drug use, my life, and my depression. I told them that every morning, I had to convince myself to stay alive one more day for my son, but didn't think I could do that for much longer.

My parents took action. To them, it was a sign of relief that I was finally asking for help and opening up. They had known for a few years something was wrong and that I wasn't doing well. But they didn't know what it was or how to help and would pray and hope every day that I would be alive in the morning. They would even have my brother drive by my house to see if I was there. They would check in with my friends to see if I seemed ok or suicidal. They even had to call the cops to check on me in fear I had taken my life. They had been suffering along with me, but the difference is I was numbing my pain, and they weren't.

The process of finding the right help wasn't an easy road. I had tried to find help in my province before, but what I found wasn't helpful. The support I needed for my mental health and addiction wasn't available. My parents began to try to navigate the system also to see if they could find help and had no luck.

But luckily my parents continued to take action. They got me into a great facility in Ontario since they could not find help in New Brunswick. We were lucky enough to have a family friend who offered to pay for the private rehab and allow us to pay it back when we were able to.

With me now in rehab in Ontario, we all started our journey to recovery. I was lucky to have such an amazing family and support system. They all embarked on the recovery journey with me so we could all heal from the emotional damage and family dysfunction addiction had brought upon us. This recovery journey has brought our family so much closer, and we have all grown so much as a result. Having my family be an open and active part of my recovery was a pivotal part of my healing from addiction.

While in rehab, I had the honor of meeting myself for the first time and getting to know the real me in the raw, without societal pressures, limiting beliefs, or masks. This was an incredible feeling that was only deepened by my newfound appreciation for meditation.

In rehab, I discovered my passion and purpose: to spread love, compassion, and hope to others suffering in silence. Little did I know that the hell I had been through would allow me to embark on this amazing journey of self-discovery, knowledge, and growth.

Three months after I got out of rehab, I started classes at Ryerson University in the mental health and addictions certification course. I crushed all my limiting beliefs that I couldn't do university because of my ADHD, or that I wasn't good at writing. Growing up, my teachers told me I couldn't write because of my bad grammar, but in University, I was able to achieve 80%-95% on most of my essays. And now I enjoy writing analogies about life and writing things such as this book.

I also enjoyed and appreciated the effects that meditation had on my life so much that I got certified to facilitate meditation and teach about the health benefits it can have on recovery and life as a whole.

Then got certified as a NADA Acudetox specialist to help others with their recovery and cravings.

I also had the opportunity to travel to Manchester, UK to get certified to facilitate mindfulness-based addiction recovery groups (MBAR) and recently co-facilitated a mindfulness retreat in Thailand with one of my mentors Valerie Mason John (author of Eight Step Recovery and co-creator of MBAR).

I am now a Certified Interventionist, certified Recovery Coach, Certified Family Recovery Coach, and trained to teach and certify other people in Canada on all three certifications with the Addictions Academy. I sit on the board for the Coalition for mental health and addiction of New Brunswick and Recovery Coaches International.

I do public speaking in communities, organizations, and schools on Mental health and addictions and do some consulting work in the addiction and recovery field.

None of this would have been possible if I was in active addiction or if I wouldn't have found myself, my passion and purpose. Now I dedicate my life to helping those suffering through addiction and their loved ones. I help them find their voice and navigate addiction and recovery.

I am passionate about doing my part in ending the stigma that is often a barrier to getting help, and in educating loved ones, and professionals about addiction and recovery. I truly believe that recovery is not only for the person going through addiction but also for the loved ones trying to help and support them.

This book was written to be a resource for family and loved ones of people going through addiction as well as for the person in active addiction or recovery. I wrote this for you to know that you are not alone, and there are resources and people out there that can help guide you through this difficult process.

There is hope!

In this book, I will give valuable information for the family and loved ones on how to love someone going through addiction without enabling them, understanding what addiction is, the importance of boundaries, their part in addiction, how to avoid codependency, and the importance of self-care in recovery.

We will also talk about the sixteen steps I use with my addiction coaching clients to support their journey to recovery. I will educate you on each step and guide you through exercises that will help you take action on each area to ultimately build a recovery lifestyle. If you are someone in active addiction, you can use this book to start your journey to recovery. If someone you love is in active addiction, you can use these steps to support them in their journey.

If you are interested in further support on the journey to a recovery lifestyle, you can find more information on my group and individualized programs by visiting www.TheRecoveryLifestyle.ca

CHAPTER 3:
ADDICTION 101

A Simplified Way to See and Understand

What everyone should know about addiction.

Addiction has been seen as a problem for a long time. It is often viewed as an incurable disease and a moral deficiency that people are powerless over. We, as a society, have taken the war on drugs approach for years and years, and we have punished people for their disease instead of helping them. This view has brought on a lot of stigma and misconceptions around addiction.

Addiction is multifaceted and complex but often is not the core issue. Addiction is usually a symptom of an underlying problem.

Addiction is a coping mechanism developed to help deal with childhood or adult trauma, difficult emotions, a loss, or a difficult situation.

If one can go back and find the root cause, they can heal from it. Then the addiction is no longer needed, and the journey to reprogramming the brain's pathways and pleasure center can begin, so the brain no longer sees the substance of choice as a necessity and reward. To heal, it is important for one to be given the space to grow and for the family and loved ones also to heal and grow. Yes, it takes time and work, but one CAN heal from addiction.

Sometimes a simple mind shift is all that is needed to give back the power and control through addiction and recovery. A simple mind shift can bring one from hopeless to hope.

This view on addiction is what I base my practice upon. But as a recovery coach, I get to meet my clients where they are at and design a custom plan for their recovery.

Because of this, I believe it's important not to be rigid in my views and recognize that every client will be different.

How and why does addiction form?

When a person feels sub-optimal for long periods, this can become their new normal. This situation can make a person susceptible to using.

If we are in this phase and decide to have a drink or use a substance, we are (even if subconsciously) doing so to feel better.

This is different than people using in an optimal frame of mind. In this case, they are using to feel good, not to feel better.

Our brain recognizes this difference. When we use to feel better, it helps us feel normal, and this triggers the reward center in our brain. This experience creates a pattern of using that feels necessary to our survival, and our ability to feel normal. We begin to need to use just like we need water, food, or air.

How to start healing from addiction?

Once we create this pattern, going without using triggers our body to give signs that we need to use or we will die. It's just like if you stop eating for seven days. After a day, your stomach will growl, then hurt, and then your mood will change your energy will be low and brain foggy, etc. All signs your body is telling you to eat, or you will die.

So, to treat the addiction, we need to start by helping people find the root cause for using as a coping mechanism. Then we can help people learn new healthier coping mechanisms, and ultimately heal from their addiction.

This sounds easy when said but finding the root cause is a difficult journey that looks different for everyone. For some, it's a lifelong journey while others can heal in a shorter period of time.

Why those going through addiction should stop trying to be sober.

To anyone silently suffering from addiction, stop seeking sobriety, and start seeking recovery.

Stop seeking the absence of your addiction, and start seeking the presence of complete health. Let's compare addiction to weight loss.

Sobriety could be compared to that new diet you started, but it never stuck.

Whereas recovery would be like implementing a healthy lifestyle. It would involve getting active, eating healthier food, surrounding yourself with positive people, etc.

Which do you think has more of a chance of sticking?

So, stop making sobriety your goal.

Because without changing your routine and way of life and without focusing your energy on healthy habits, you're setting yourself up for a more challenging and difficult journey. Instead, choose to walk the path to recovery.

Instead, you can choose: - A new way of life, - New healthy routines - Cooking and eating good food - Meeting new and positive people - Focusing your time and energy on you - Finding joy and happiness.

When you make your goal complete health, a new you can and will emerge. When you see the big picture, you simplify the journey. Ultimately, when you make your goal recovery, sobriety will follow.

The role of perception in addiction recovery.

Perception is a very important and powerful tool we have as human beings. Often, we end up causing our suffering with our perception of things, situations, or people. We make up stories, positive or negative, that are not facts, but we treat them as such.

Two people can witness an event or meet the same person, or go through something emotional, and both perceive the same situation differently.

How the situation is perceived will help determine the effect it has on us. The length of time we stay attached to our perception of the situation will help decide how long we keep ourselves in a state of suffering.

Knowing this, why not be mindful of our perception and consciously choose to perceive things in the most positive way possible?

Adjusting our perception is not about lying to ourselves or avoiding the issues or reality. No, it's about making better choices on what thoughts or beliefs we will feed our brain. Yes, I agree, not all situations are positive, good, or happy, but it's about choosing to see the positive in even the hardest situations. It's about understanding that most events or emotions in our life are NOT permanent. As hard as it might be, if we find the positive aspects of the learning experience associated with the event or situation, we can help minimize the pain, negative brain chatter, and negative outcomes. Instead, we can shorten the suffering period and use it to learn and grow as a person.

Example:

Limiting thought: "I'm having such a bad day!!"

Questions to ask: Are you having a bad day? The whole day? Or did you have a bad moment or event?

In that example, having the perception we are having a bad day will help propel us towards having a bad day because we are holding on to that perception.

In reality, maybe we had a bad moment in the day, and we can acknowledge "what just happened sucked, but I won't let it affect my day," or we can say to ourselves "wow that hurt but what can I learn from it?" and then do something to get our mind off it and continue to enjoy our day.

Here's a great way to reframe your perception on every situation in your life:

- What do I have control over in this situation?

- Have I done my part in taking action on things I have control over?

- If you answer yes to both the above, then accepting that you have no more control over the situation is important. This will allow you to put it aside and focus on the rest of your day in places your time and energy will have a positive impact on your life.

WANT TO EXPERIENCE WHAT IT'S LIKE TO RECOVER FROM ADDICTION?

Try the 7 Day Sugar-Free Challenge

The best way to get a glimpse as to what it can feel like to be going through addiction is to give up an addictive substance you probably already consume-Sugar.

I challenge you to start today for the next seven days: no sugar, no carbs, no fruits, no artificial or natural sugars.

Then journal your moods and emotions, body changes or aches, messages your body is sending you as well as note triggers you encounter that give you an urge to have sugar or quit the challenge.

Going through this challenge will likely be hard, but overcoming a drug or substance addiction is about 10x harder. This exercise will give you compassion for the hard work it takes to overcome substance addiction

Find a template for journaling your sugar-free experience on the following pages.

*If you already live a sugar-free life, go seven days without caffeine or electronics.

I'd love to hear about your experience with the seven-day sugar challenge.

Email me at info@nevergiveuphope.ca if you'd like to share your experience.

Sugar-Free Challenge exercise courtesy of Dr. Cali Estes and The Addictions Academy.

PART TWO:

UNDERSTANDING ADDICTION & THE FAMILY'S ROLE IN RECOVERY

CHAPTER 4: CODEPENDENCY

What is codependency, and why is it dangerous?

How is codependency defined?

Claudia Black defines Codependency as: "an emotional disorder that causes someone to ignore their own needs while feeling compelled to fulfill the needs of others. He or she may forfeit their own well-being and values in pursuit of pleasing other people."

In other words, it's trying to help someone that doesn't want help, or trying to help someone even if it affects our health or life negatively. It's putting our own life aside and focusing all our energy and time on helping someone else despite the negative impact it's having on us. Ultimately, it is living our life for someone else.

Codependency and Addiction

When someone is in active addiction, there is often codependency that develops in a family system. The person going through the addiction often becomes codependent on a loved one to cover up for them or enable them so they can use. Also, often, one or more of the loved ones become codependent on helping the person going through the addiction. Their whole life starts revolving around the person going through the addiction. They spend a lot of their time trying thinking about how to help them, how to protect them, and how to find excuses for them, so they don't lose their jobs or reputation. After a while the loved one gets lost in this pattern and lifestyle and loses themselves. Their self-worth now depends on their role as the helper or protector of the one going through the addiction.

As a loved one, it's important to recognize your part is in the addiction and if codependency has sneaked up. If it has, it is very important to get on the recovery journey whether or not the loved one going through the addiction decides to recover or not. This will be a big step in modeling recovery and self-care to your loved one who is suffering.

How can you identify if you have a codependent relationship?

- Have I covered or lied for my loved one who is in active addiction?

- Have I stopped my hobbies to support my loved one in active addiction?

- Have I lost interest in things I use to love to make time to help my loved one in active addiction?

- Does my world revolve around my loved one in active addiction?

- Do I have clear boundaries to protect myself, my health, and mental wellbeing? Do I still take time for myself for self-care and self-love?

Answer the questions on the previous page honestly to yourself, and if you think there might be codependency in your family system, take the first step, and seek professional help to heal from the effects. This is a great step towards helping your loved one get out of addiction by modeling recovery and gaining knowledge on addiction and how to heal your family.

If the family starts healing, it will make the healing process easier for the loved one in active addiction.

CHAPTER 5:
ENABLING VS LOVING

Learning how to support a loved one in active addiction instead of enabling

When supporting a loved one through addiction it can be very hard to walk the line between enabling and loving.

This chapter is dedicated to showing you how to love someone in active addiction without slipping into potentially dangerous enabling behaviors.

When someone is in active addiction, their focus is on three things:

1. Finding their next fix

2. Using

3. Hiding that they've used

This will often lead to lies manipulation to accomplish their perceived need for using.

It can be hard as a loved one to figure out what's true and what's false.

"Am I being manipulated, or is it a need?"

Because of this, we often end up enabling our loved one that is going through the addiction.

Our intentions are good, but the result is we end up enabling them.

This can have a very negative impact. It prolongs the time it would naturally take to hit their rock bottom and thus can make the rock bottom more severe.

The longer it takes to hit rock bottom and get help, the more chances of jail, death, or irreversible effects on the brain and body.

To help your loved one in their recovery, you must learn the difference between enabling and loving by showing support.

SO, WHAT'S THE DIFFERENCE?

Enabling

Helping with or doing something for your loved one they should be doing themselves.

Ex. Helping a loved one do their groceries or paying for them.

Supporting

You are helping or doing something for your loved one that they can't do by themselves.

Ex. Helping a loved one carry their luggage because it's too heavy for them or because they have a back issue that prevents them from doing it.

How to Show Love Without Enabling

This can be tricky because we often feel guilt or shame for what our loved one is going through and blame ourselves. Well, let me tell you it's not your fault! The past is in the past, and we have no control over it, but we do have control over our actions today, and we need act out of common sense and best welfare for our loved one in active addiction not react out of emotion because we feel guilty. Stopping the enabling and replacing it with love and support will be a big step in everyone's recovery.

What enabling looks like

- Giving money
- Paying their bills
- Giving clothes or food
- Allowing to live at home for free
- Bailing them out of jail or trouble
- Making excuses for their behavior
- Making excuses for missing work or school
- not having boundaries
- not enforcing boundaries

What supporting looks like

- Telling them you love them often
- Letting them know you are there when they are ready to get help
- Inviting them for a family dinner
- Having clear boundaries
- Enforcing boundaries and consequences
- Helping find treatment or therapy
- Helping pay for treatment or therapy
- Being present if the loved one needs to talk about their emotions or hardships

Going from enabling to being supportive can seem and feel difficult. And often it is, but keep in mind when you're enabling, you're helping your loved one to slowly kill themselves. When you're supporting, you're observing them on their journey offering love. You are also choosing to be ready to fully support them when they do ask for help.

It's important for all loved ones to make an inventory of how they have enabled in the past and how they are still enabling. Then to make a plan to stop enabling and set clear boundaries with the loved one to prevent future enabling. You can use the grid found on TheRecoveryLifestyle.ca website to get a visual on your enabling behavior and how you can transform them into supportive.

How to Prevent Manipulation

A good way to prevent being manipulated by a loved one going through the addiction is to try to always speak to him or her in teams of two.

This can be very important in early recovery or if the person is still in active addiction. It's much harder to manipulate two people at the same time.

CHAPTER 6: RELAPSE, LAPSE, AND SIGNS OF USE

How to recognize and move on from relapse or lapse in recovery

Using Lapses or Relapses as a Learning Experience

It's important to remember that addiction is a learned behavior or coping mechanism and that sobriety is also a learned behavior. It's important to be patient and supportive, allowing our loved one time and space to learn the new behavior and reprogram old ones.

In the event of a Relapse or a Lapse (slip), our perception of that incident will have a big impact on our loved one that is suffering through addiction. A relapse or Lapse can be used as a positive learning experience and should be viewed that way.

When relapse or lapse occurs, our loved one does not forget everything he or she has learned about recovery, but it does provide a real-life situation that can be used to learn from and grow to strengthen recovery.

But if the relapse or lapse is dealt with like a negative event, our loved one will feel shame and guilt. This can trigger long term relapse or make the recovery process longer and more painful for everyone. So as long as the person going through the addiction can take the time to understand why they lapsed or relapsed the event can be positive.

What is a Relapse?

When someone goes back to their old addictive behaviors or substance use for some time without considerations of the effects it is having on their health, social life, and people around them.

What is a Lapse (Slip)?

When someone has a moment of confusion and uses there substance or substitutes with another substance, but realizes this is wrong and gets back on track with their recovery.

A lapse can easily turn into relapse without the proper support and non-judgmental environment.

Three Stages of Relapse?

1. Emotional Relapse

The first stage of relapse and usually happens before the person even thinks about using. We can see this in the persons change of moods, emotions, eating, and sleeping habits. This is often brought on or amplified by the lack of, or decline in using their support system and learned strategies. If we can identify the relapse in this stage, we can prevent the mental and physical relapse.

2. Mental Relapse

The second stage of relapse is where "stinking thinking" get out of control. It becomes an internal battle in their mind. One part is happy to be sober the other part fantasizes about using again. We can notice this stage when our loved one starts talking about the good old days when they used or talking about maybe it could be possible to use again. Once our loved one had mentally decided they will use its only a matter of time before they have a physical relapse and use.

3. Physical Relapse

This stage is what most of us think about when we hear relapse. It's when the person decides to and uses again. Using one time can bring on intense cravings to continue using. Getting your loved one back on track to recovery or in treatment is very important at this stage. It can be a great learning experience that can strengthen their recovery or a deal-breaker that brings them back into active addiction. The way we react to the physical relapse makes all the difference.

Creating a relapse prevention plan

Having a good solid relapse prevention plan in place is crucial to the recovery process.

Your relapse prevention plan is personal to you, and we will create this later in the book.

This is also something I go over in-depth with my clients in my 8-week group recovery program.

Warning Signs for Each of the Three Stages of Relapse

Emotional Relapse

- Change in moods

- Difficulty with emotion regulation

- Change in sleep habits

- Change eating habits

- Lack of motivation

- Signs of depression

- Stopping or changing hobbies

- Anger when questioned

- Feeling overwhelmed

Mental Relapse

- Romanticizing about using
- Start hanging with old friends that use
- Talking about the ability to use
- Diminishing effects addiction had
- Finding excuses or rationalizing the possibility of using
- Good habits that help recovery are left aside
- No more talk about recovery

Physical Relapse

- Loss of weight
- Loss of appetite
- Isolation
- Loss of passion for life and activities
- Change in behavior
- Change in hygiene
- Change in how they dress
- Change in friends
- Avoids discussion on recovery

- Avoids eye contact

- Visibly more anxious or fidgety

- Lies and manipulation

- Issues with job or finances

CHAPTER 7:
NOT ALL REHABS ARE
CREATED EQUAL

Finding a rehab that is the right fit can make or break the recovery process

Finding the right rehab

Often a big step in the recovery process is finding a suitable rehab for our loved one. This is where things often go wrong. We often think all rehabs are created equal, and that any will do.

Unfortunately, this is not the case. There is a lot to consider when it comes to choosing the right rehab facility.

Because addiction is multi-faceted and not a one size fits all solution, it's important that the process of choosing a rehab reflects the person going through addiction. Over the years, various type of rehabs using different philosophies, techniques, and strategies have popped up. This is great if you know what to look for and how to choose the right rehab for your loved one's needs.

For example, if your loved one is not religious or is pushed away by faith, the last thing we want to do is send them to a faith-based rehab. There are already enough barriers to the vulnerability required to dig deep and find the root of the addiction; the last thing we want to do is add a wall or barrier to that journey.

Questions to ask which will help you figure out the best rehab for your loved one.

- Does he or she believe in a higher power?

- Does he or she believe in religion?

- Does he or she believe in energy healing?

- Does he or she believe in alternative medicine?

- Have they been to treatment before? If yes, how many times and where?

- Does he or she self-harm? Have they ever self-harmed? When's the last time?

- Is he or she suicidal? Have they attempted suicide? If so, when?

- Does he or she have any known or suspected mental health conditions?

- Does he or she have a history of being aggressive or violent?

- What's their drug of choice? How long have they been using?

- Does he or she have any special talents or passions?

- Would he or she be ok with a hospital setting or require more of a residential setting?

- Any history of abuse or past trauma?

- What are their hobbies?

- Is he or she on probation or have any criminal charges?

- Is he or she high profile (CEO, celebrity, or public figure)?

- Is he or she front line responders (police, firefighter, doctor, pilot, etc.)?

- Do they have insurance coverage for rehab? If not, what is their budget for rehab?

Services offered by rehabs

The questions on the previous page are important to help find a rehab with the right approach for your loved one. The next area to consider when choosing a rehab are what services they offer, and how they will meet the needs of your loved one.

Below is a list of types of treatment with a description to help you navigate the treatment types and terms.

- **DETOX** *often 7-9 days* – Remove substance from the system and/or set up medication management program.

- **RESIDENTIAL REHAB INPATIENT** 28-30 days min, no max stay – Typically involves self-discovery, a structured environment, support 24/7, learning strategies to stay sober, group and one on one therapy.

- **RECOVERY COACH** Custom Timeline – Works on present and future, not on past. A strength-based approach that helps find the passion and set goals for life and recovery. Can help with abstinent based recovery or harm reduction.

- **HALFWAY OR SOBER HOUSE** Min 1 month recommended 3-6 months – Involves a zero-tolerance sober living arrangement with drug testing.

- **PARTIAL HOSPITALIZATION** Often 5 days a week for 30 days – Involves day treatment where the patient undergoes group therapy, one on one therapy, and other services. They go to treatment all day then go home for the evenings.

- **INTENSIVE OUTPATIENT PROGRAM** Often six weeks, 3x a week, for 3 hours – Involves part-time treatment often including but not limited to group therapy and one on one therapy.

- **SUPPORT GROUPS** Free and can attend meetings as desired – Often a 12 step or 8 step recovery group. With group support, often complete sobriety is the goal. Group support also typically involves sponsorship.

- **SOBER COMPANION** for a specific event or predetermined amount of time – Kind of like a sitter, stays with the person for a determined period or for a specific event to help make good choices and stay on track with recovery.

*Descriptions adapted from the Recovery Coach training from the Addictions Academy.
www.TheAddictionsAcademy.com

CHAPTER 8:
THE IMPORTANCE OF SELF-CARE

Self-care is not just for the person going through addiction; it's for the entire family.

Self-care is not only for your loved one who is going through addiction or in recovery. Self-care is very important for the whole family, and it's a great way to model recovery for our loved one.

When a loved one is in active addiction, the whole family often loses themselves trying to help. So, it is crucial to take your life back and give ourselves the honor and love of finding yourselves, finding your passions, and doing things for yourself again.

It's important to rebuild a life that revolves around your welfare and best interest, not the welfare of others.

If you've lost yourself helping someone you love, it can be hard to refocus your time and energy on yourself. Here are a few tricks to help you get started:

- Write a list of things you use to love doing but don't seem to find time to do anymore or just stopped doing completely.

- Write a bucket list and start making plans to accomplish them.

- Reserve 1 hour/day for the most important person in your life, YOU. Just relax and enjoy life.

- Reconnect with old friends and don't turn down an opportunity to re-connect and do activities with friends.

- Find a new hobby you've always wanted to try and do it.

- Start a gratitude list every day.

- Make self-care a priority in your life (walking, meditation, yoga, a massage, watching sports, getting nails done, etc.)

Remember you're the most important person in your life, love yourself and care for yourself because if you get sick or burned out, then you can no longer help others and will struggle to help yourself. So, fill your glass first, then you can pour into other people's cup.

PART THREE:

THE 16 STEP METHOD TO CREATING A RECOVERY LIFESTYLE

A note from André about implementing a Recovery Lifestyle.

The following section is dedicated to helping you or your loved one with implementing the essentials for building a Recovery Lifestyle.

There are 16 core elements to a Recovery Lifestyle, and I am going to teach you about each, and offer exercises to help you implement them.

Each chapter in this section will include information and an explanation of each step to a recovery lifestyle, and a series of questions or an action to take to apply it to your life.

Don't skip the activities and questions. This is where the real progress will occur. Take the time to apply this to your life, or to support someone you love in applying it in theirs.

The results of implementing a recovery lifestyle are incredible, and I am excited to hear more about your journey with implementing your own.

Sincerely,
André

CHAPTER 9:
FINDING YOUR PASSION

**Because passion gives us a
reason to wake up every day.**

Finding our passion is the first step in creating your recovery lifestyle.

The reason this is such an important first step is that being in active addiction becomes your purpose. Finding and using your substance of choice becomes the most important thing in your life. It becomes the thing for which you strive.

But once we decide to stop using and create a new healthy recovery lifestyle, it's common to feel bored. We no longer wake up to the same purpose. Same goes with the family or loved ones that have someone going through addiction. We often put our passions aside to tend to our loved one and end up forgetting about ourselves and what we love in the process.

So, when the loved one gets on the path of recovery, we are often left with a void. So, in both cases, it is crucial to find our passion.

What are you passionate about, and how can you align yourself with that passion? This will help everyone ease anxiety and have direction. And having a clear direction will help guide healthy and positive decisions.

Why is finding your passion important?

- Because passion is like the light from a lighthouse: if you see it and follow it, you will find your way.

- Having a passion gives us reason to wake up every day.

- Finding your passion helps you make better choices to achieve your passion.

- Finding your passion helps with our self-worth and confidence.

- Finding your passion can help with anxiety and the uncertainty of what the future holds.

- Remember, a dream is only a dream unless you make an action plan to make it a reality.

Finding Your Passion Exercise

List 5 things you used to enjoy before:

1.

2.

3.

4.

5.

Now circle the top three you still find interesting or intriguing

For each one, you circled write down 3-5 things needed for you to be able to enjoy this again.

1.	1.	1.
2.	2.	2.
3.	3.	3.
4.	4.	4.
5.	5.	5.

Now let's create a bucket list. Come up with a list of the top ten things you'd be proud to do or accomplish in the next five years. What would excite you to get to do?

1.

2.

3.

4.

5.

6.

7.

8.

9.

10.

Now circle the top 5 you'd like to accomplish. Then highlight the top 5 easiest to accomplish.

Look at the ones that have been circled and highlighted and focus on those to start.

For each item that is both circled and highlighted, list three things you need to accomplish to reach that goal, and when you will take action.

Goal #1

First Steps	Action Date
1.	1.
2.	2.
3.	3.

Goal #2

First Steps	Action Date
1.	1.
2.	2.
3.	3.

Goal #3

First Steps	Action Date
1.	1.
2.	2.
3.	3.

CHAPTER 10:
MENTAL WELLNESS

**Creating resilient mental
health to support your recovery.**

What is mental wellness, and why does it matter?

Mind fitness is about how healthy and resilient your brain is, and about the tools you have to improve and manage your mental health.

Our brain is the most important organ in our body, yet it's the organ we tend to the least. It's also the organ with which we have the most shame and stigma around getting help.

We need to change how we see caring for our brain in society. It should be one of the most important organs to care for, and if we care for our brain, we are automatically caring for our whole body.

For example, if we have a hard time seeing we go to an optometrist, if we have a cough or fever we go to the doctor, a toothache we go to the dentist. With all other parts of the body, we take action and seek help when something is wrong. But if we have difficulty with our thoughts, emotions, trauma, mental health issues, or addiction, we are ashamed and feel the stigma, so we avoid seeking help. This only intensifies our struggle.

So let's break the stigma, love our bodies including our brain and lets all work together to make seeing a therapist, counselor, coach, psychiatrist or doctor part of the norm and part of our normal yearly checkup.

Let's educate our families and loved ones struggling with addiction to strategies, techniques, and routines that will help care for our brains. Because we all deserve the opportunity and ability to care for our brains as much as we care for the rest of our body.

Tools and Strategies to Help with Mental Wellness

- Meditation (5-10 min/day to start)

- Eating healthy (your gut health has a big impact on your brain.

- Exercise and physical activity (proven to help regulate mood and help in recovery)

- Talking with someone you trust to open up about feelings and struggles.

- Hobbies that bring joy

- Self-care every day

- Reading or educating yourself

What is meditation, and why is it important for recovery?

There are many definitions as to what meditation is, please feel free to read up on those. But this is how I explain Meditation to beginners:

Meditation is about spending some time alone with yourself without judging yourself or your thoughts.

How can meditation support recovery?

Meditation helps keep the balance between your Sympathetic (Fight, Flight, Freeze) and Parasympathetic (rest and restore) systems. With evolution our stressors have changed. In the caveman era the system was very well designed. Most of the time, people are in the Parasympathetic mode unless they are in danger, or are being attacked by predators.

But today with all the digital stressors we have created as a society (internet, cellphones, cars, etc.) we now spend most of our time in the sympathetic mode. This causes anxiety, depression, addiction, and many other illnesses because our body doesn't go into Parasympathetic mode as much as needed to rest and restore so our body and mind can heal itself and balance all functions.

This is why it's so important to develop strategies like meditation that allow us to go into Parasympathetic mode and restore and rest.

Common Meditation Misconceptions

#1: You must clear your mind of all thoughts, or you must not have any thoughts.

For most, having zero thoughts is not realistic, and truly if you're a beginner having zero thoughts shouldn't be your goal.

Meditation is about spending some time alone with yourself without judging yourself or your thoughts. We spend all day judging ourselves and wagging the finger at ourselves "I shouldn't have said that, I will never get this right, why do I always do this, I don't like the way I look, etc." But in meditation, we spend time loving ourselves in a non-judgmental way.

Accepting that we will have thoughts is important. It's what we do with the thoughts that matters. When a thought arises don't judge it, it's a thought, neither good or bad. We let it pass and bring our attention back to our breath.

The more we do this, the easier it gets, and the more we do it, the fewer thoughts that will arise.

Everyone deserves the opportunity and honor to sit with themselves and be with themselves in a non-judgmental way.

#2: You must sit in a proper meditation position to meditate, or you must follow certain meditation rules and guidelines.

False, the beautiful thing about meditation is that it's a personal practice, and there are no rules.

You meditate in the area and position with which you feel comfortable. As long as you can give yourself the opportunity to meditate daily, the technique or position won't matter, you'll still get benefits from the practice.

Now with that said, after you start feeling comfortable with your meditation practice, I would invite you to do some research into various positions and guidelines that can help amplify your meditation.

But to start the important thing to remember is making meditation part of your daily routine and giving yourself the love of spending time in silence with yourself without judgment.

#3: You must meditate for long periods. (30 minutes or more)

If you're a beginner and set the expectation of meditating for 30 minutes from the start, you're setting yourself up for disappointment.

The best advice I can give you is to never go into a meditation with expectations. Go into meditation with an open mind and no times restraints or expectations of any outcome.

If you start and end up meditating for 5 minutes, that's great. Keep meditating, and with time and practice, you will realize your meditations will grow longer and longer.

When will you meditate?

Pick a time of day and stick to it!

I will meditate during _____ time of the day.

Three guided meditations to use to get started.

The 3 Minute Meditation - Adapted from a meditation learned from Valerie Mason John

A simple 3-minute meditation to help bring you to the present moment so you can make clear-minded decisions and regulate your emotions

Get in a comfortable position. Close your eyes softly — breathe in through your nostrils and out thru your nostrils.

Take three deep breaths in and out. If any thoughts arise know that it's ok, don't judge them just let them pass and gently bring your attention back to your breath (in-out)

On your next few inhales, imagine/visualize or feel the breath going thru your body down to your feet. Feel your feet touching the floor; try to feel your socks or shoes between your feet and the floor.

On your next few inhales, imagine/visualize or feel the breath going through your body down to your thighs, feel your hand or arms resting on your thighs, feel your clothing between your thigh and your arms or hands.

On your next few inhales, imagine/visualize or feel the breath going through your body down to your butt. Feel your butt touching the chair; try to feel your clothing between your butt and the chair.

On your next few inhales, imagine/visualize or feel the breath going through your body down to your back. Feel your back touching the chair; try to feel your clothing between your back and the chair.

On your next few inhales, imagine/visualize or feel the breath going to your head. Feel your hair on your head. Glasses on your face or hair touching your forehead.

On your next few inhales, imagine/visualize or feel the breath going through your nostrils. Feel the breath tickling your upper lip as it goes in and out.

Take three deep breath, and then when you are ready, slowly bring your attention back to the room. Wiggle your toes and fingers. And enjoy your day.

A Sleep Meditation - Created by Jivasu, creator of the Naturality program.

This meditation will help you get a good night's rest and help you peacefully fall asleep

The night meditation technique has four parts to it.

1. Sleep pose: Lie in bed on your right side, with your hands touching and ankle or legs crossed over each other.

2. Letting go of the day: Remember the day (visual, feelings, touch, smell, taste and sounds) in reverse order starting slowly from the last event of the day and reaching to the point where you just woke up from the sleep in the morning.

3. Deep breathing: Take seven deep sleep relaxing breaths.

4. Light in heart: Visualize, imagine or feel a flame or light in the middle of two eyebrows. Slowly allow it to descend along the midline of nose, lips, chin, and neck to establish deep in heart space in the middle of the chest. Remain focused on it and gently slip into sleep.

A Self-Love Medication - Created by Jivasu, creator of the Naturality program.

For times when you are feeling down about yourself, or your recovery progress, you can use this meditation to self-soothe.

Sitting comfortably in a chair or on the floor, remember some moments when your body and mind were filled with love and affection.

You are not an observer or these moments but are reliving them. You are feeling the love and affection of those moments, here and now.

Allow that love and affection to fill you and to flow from head to toe.

This feeling of love and affection is filling your:

- headspace
- eyes face, jaw, mouth
- ear
- neck

- chest

- abdomen

- left shoulder, upper arm, elbow, forearm, wrist, hand, fingers, and thumb

- right shoulder, upper arm, elbow, forearm, wrist, hand, thumb, and finger

- upper, middle and lower back

- pelvic area

- left hip, thigh, knee, leg, ankle, foot and toes

- right hip, thigh, knee, leg, ankle, foot and toes

- emotions and thoughts

You also remember any words, sound, aroma, taste, and touch that were present in those moments. Allow your whole being to merge into that feeling of love.

Now feel the energy of love and affection in your body, particularly in the area of your heart.

Allow the energy in your body and heart to flow towards your hands, fingers, and thumbs. Your hands, fingers, and thumbs are vibrating with loving energy.

With your hands, fingers, and thumbs, slowly and tenderly touch, and gently press:

- the sides of your head

- your eyes your face, jaw, and ears

- your neck

- your shoulders, upper arm, elbows, forearm, hands, fingers, and thumbs

- your chest

- your abdomen

- your pelvic area

- your thighs, knee, legs, ankle, feet, and toes

- the parts of your back accessible to you

- your first chakra at the base of your spine

- your second chakra just above your pubic bone

- your third chakra at your naval area

- your fourth chakra in the middle of your chest

- your fifth chakra at the root of your neck

- your sixth chakra in the middle of two eyebrows

- your seventh chakra on the top of your head

Your mental wellness checkup.

What are you doing to take care of and improve your mental health?

What could you be doing to improve your mental health?

Choose five things you will start doing to better improve your mental health:

CHAPTER 11:
SOUL FITNESS

Creating strong soul guiding principles.

What is soul fitness?

Soul fitness is about having a healthy belief system and guiding principles for your life.

What are beliefs?

Having a belief system is very important to recovery. It relieves stress, and it helps to trust that something or someone is looking out for us. It could be a higher power, religion, meditation, the universe, the stars, the moon or sun, or even trees. It doesn't matter, as long as you believe in something.

What are guiding principles?

Guiding principles are the guidelines you use to direct your life. The guidelines that you base your decisions on. The guidelines that represent who you are and what you stand for.

Guiding Principles Exercise

Using the following page as inspiration, write down a list of 10 guiding principles you want to live your life by.

GUIDING PRINCIPLES INSPIRATION

- In life, I will give more than I take
- My time is more valuable than money
- I live beneath my means
- I accept that life isn't fair
- I do nice things and try not to get caught
- I listen more and talk less
- I walk for 30 minutes every day
- My family is always my priority
- I choose not to worry about money
- If it doesn't matter in 5 years, I won't spend more than 5 minutes being upset about it.
- I see failure as a beginning, not an end
- If I never go after it, I won't have it
- I always do more than is expected of me
- I invest my time teaching others
- I do work that matters to me

Write down ten guiding principles that inspire you and challenge you to want to be the person you want to be.

1.

2.

3.

4.

5.

6.

7.

8.

9.

10.

Now narrow these down to three to five principles that truly inspire you. Cut these out or write them down on a piece of paper to put in your wallet. Use them as a reference with every decision you make.

CHAPTER 12: GRATITUDE

How to rewire your brain for more positive thinking.

Gratitude is defined as by Angeles Arrien in her book *Living in Gratitude: A Journey That Will Change Your Life*, as follows:

"Gratitude is a feeling that spontaneously emerges from within. However, it is not simply an emotional response; it is also a choice we make. We can choose to be grateful, or we can choose to be ungrateful — to take our gifts and blessings for granted. As a choice, gratitude is an attitude or disposition."

As writer Alexis de Tocqueville once described it, gratitude is:

"A habit of the heart."

Brother Davide Steindl-Rast, a Benedictine monk, reminds us that:

"Gratefulness is the inner gesture of giving meaning to our life by receiving life as a gift."

M. J. Ryan's classic book, *Attitudes of Gratitude*, supports the idea that gratitude is a stance we voluntarily take, and one we can adopt through the difficult seasons of life as well as the good ones.

"The daily practice of gratitude keeps the heart open, regardless of what comes our way."

In active addiction, we can end up having many negative experiences and with time have less and less hope. Our view on life and the world, in general, becomes darker, and we tend to overlook the positive things that remain in our lives.

Same goes with families and loved ones of the person going through the addiction. Our pain of seeing someone we love slowly killing themselves can lead us to not seeing the positive things in our life.

Incorporating the simple exercise at the end of this chapter can help in a very subtle way to rewire our brains into seeing and appreciating the positive instead of going directly to all that negative. This can have a huge impact on our recovery and on creating our recovery lifestyle.

Gratitude Exercise

Gratitude is so important because it helps rewire our brain to positive thinking and feelings.

Every day write down a list of 3-5 things for which you are grateful.

Today I am grateful for...

1.

2.

3.

4.

5.

Today I am proud of myself for...

1.

2.

CHAPTER 13:
NUTRITION

How to use nutrition to positively impact your recovery.

As mentioned previously, nutrition and gut health are very important to brain health and physical health. So, in this section, we will look at foods that can help in recovery and foods or habits that can impact our recovery in a negative way.

Again, recovery is a lifestyle, so we have to create a good lifestyle to facilitate our recovery. As a family, it's important to model this for our loved one going through addiction, but it's also very important for our health.

What you eat can impact your recovery positively or negatively depending on the choices you make. One common mistake we often make in early recovery is to not focus on our diet and our gut. What we eat changes how we feel, it can affect our moods, energy, and how our body heals.

In active addiction we damage our insides in many ways, often our gut can be damaged (leaky gut) this makes it hard for our body to absorb the nutrients we need from the food we eat. Our hormones can be out of balance, and we can also be deficient in nutrients. All this can be part of what causes our brain to feel foggy or our energy to be low. Certain foods or ingredients can be very beneficial to help our bodies heal, but some can be very negative and can be a danger for relapse.

Two foods that we often turn to in recovery are Sugar and Caffeine; both of these foods we should stay away from. Sugar and caffeine both give us the rush of dopamine we crave and pursued with drugs. With sugar and caffeine, we get the fast high and quick crash we got with drugs, and this can lead to a more depressed state in return can lead to relapse.

Also, one of the goals in recovery is to help create new healthy pathways in the brain to heal from the addiction. By exposing ourselves to caffeine and sugar, it makes it harder and takes longer to create those new pathways since we keep engaging in instant gratification with quick high and then come down.

> *Head on over to www.TheRecoveryLifestyle.ca and join our Book Club! You'll receive a detailed Addiction Recovery Food & Meal Plan designed to support your recovery success!*

Common Health issues of people who have been through addiction:

- Leaky Gut, not absorbing nutrients properly

- Deficiencies in Amino Acids, Minerals and Vitamins, low energy, foggy brain, weight management issues, emotional regulation.

- Low blood sugar can be part of the cause of depression, anxiety, and panic attacks.

Common Amino Acids, Minerals, and Vitamins deficiencies include:

- Tyrosine, the precursor to the "feel good" neurotransmitter dopamine.

  Associated with:

  o Low energy, low motivation, depressed mood, intense cravings

- L-glutamine, an amino acid with immune and antioxidant benefits.

  Associated with:

  o Can help reduce sugar cravings. Sugar consumption is linked to higher rates of anxiety, depression, and inflammation.

    o Boost immune cell activity in the gut, and this helps prevent infection. Heal the gut.

    o Help with inflammation in the gut and soothes the gut.

- Antioxidants, help to rebuild your immune system in the aftermath and also can help speed up the body's cleansing and regeneration process.

- GABA, the main inhibitory neurotransmitter in the brain the promotes calm and relaxation.

Associated with:

    o Less brain fog, better cognition, better sleep

- Tryptophan is an essential amino acid and a precursor to serotonin.

Associated with:

    o Positive, happy mood.

- Vitamins that might be depleted: Vitamin B, C, D, Magnesium

Foods that support recovery

- Whole Foods
- Vegetables
- Fruits
- Gluten-free oatmeal
- Sprouted rice, Jasmine or Basmati
- Avocado
- Nuts
- Organic Poultry (L-Glutamine, tyrosine)
- Organic Fish (L-Glutamine, tyrosine)
- Organic Meat (L-Glutamine, tyrosine)
- Turkey, Lamb, Pork (tryptophan, tyrosine)
- Banana (tyrosine)
- Sunflower seeds (tyrosine)
- Soybeans (tyrosine)
- Eggs (L-Glutamine)
- Kale (L-Glutamine)
- Spinach (L-Glutamine)
- Parsley (L-Glutamine)
- Beets (L-Glutamine)
- Carrots (L-Glutamine)
- Brussel sprouts (L-Glutamine)

- Beans (L-Glutamine)
- Papaya (L-Glutamine)
- Blueberries
- Strawberries (antioxidants)
- Leaks (antioxidants)
- Pecans (antioxidants)
- Artichokes (antioxidants)
- Onions (antioxidants)
- Kefir (GABA)
- Shrimp (GABA)
- Cherry tomatoes (GABA)
- Lentils (tryptophan)
- Oat Brand (tryptophan)
- Coconut oil
- Flaxseed

Foods that detract from recovery

- Sugar
- Caffeine
- Dairy
- Processed foods
- Additives or preservatives
- White flour

- Hydrogenated and refined fats
- Margarine
- Shortening
- Artificial coloring
- High fructose corn syrup
- Dextrose
- Aspartame
- MSG
- Phosphates
- Tobacco

Meal plan and nutrition information courtesy of Dr. Renée Purdy.

CHAPTER 14:
RANDOM ACTS OF KINDNESS

Building self-worth through actions focused on others.

Random acts of kindness are good for many reasons, but the two primary ones are:

1. It's a great way to give back to the community and help others.

2. It helps us feel better about ourselves and build a stronger sense of self-worth.

So, as part of your recovery lifestyle, integrate and be mindful about doing at least 1 act of kindness every day. It can be as simple as opening a door for someone, smiling at someone, giving someone a compliment, paying it forward at a coffee shop, or helping an elderly to carry their groceries.

This might seem insignificant, but from experience, I've seen this exercise help people in many ways. I've seen this help some clients get the feel-good feeling they needed to get past a struggle they were going through that day all while bringing love and light to someone else in need.

I've seen families doing this activity together and have seen some pretty amazing outcomes come from this. It's helped families get closer and strengthen their family bond. In return, the act of kindness helped someone plus helped the process of healing the family system.

Your task: every day, perform one random act of kindness.

CHAPTER 15:
YOUR BAG OF INFLUENCE

Building a strong and loving support system.

Your bag of influence is a list of people that are part of your life. Whether you are in active addiction, started the journey to a healthy recovery lifestyle, in recovery, or a loved one supporting someone going through addiction, this exercise will help you discover who is a positive influence in your life and who is not as positive.

With this knowledge, you can choose to spend more time with the positive influences and supports and less with the not so positive supports.

Who you surround yourself with can have a major impact on your recovery lifestyle and family system success or failure. Please fill out the following page with your influences.

Who has been an influence on your life in the following timelines?

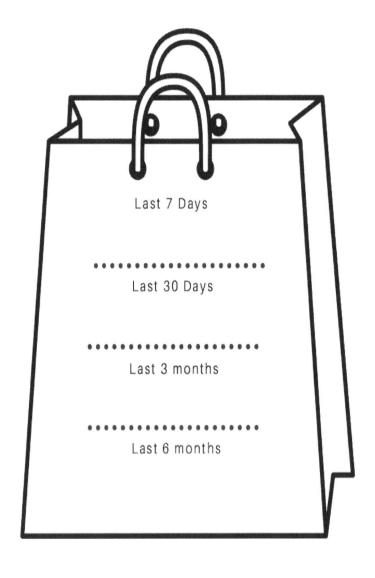

Last 7 Days

· ·

Last 30 Days

· ·

Last 3 months

· ·

Last 6 months

- Now in your bag, highlight the names that are in more than one row.

- Now circle the people that have a positive influence on your life.

- Now mark an X next to people that are a negative influence

- Now mark a checkmark next to those with whom you have used.

If you're like most people, your bag is probably too heavy and in danger of collapsing.

Metaphorically speaking, your life might be too full with outside negativity or triggers or people that drain your energy and put you at danger of relapse.

Take time to look at your bag, do you have anyone that is highlighted and has a circle around with no checks or X's? These are the light items that your bag can handle and will be beneficial to you. If yes, write them down here:

These people should at the top of your bag of influence, and continuing a relationship and creating a connection with them is important.

Now write all the ones with a circle and no X's or checks:

These people should also be part of your close friends and in the box of influence.

Now write all those that have an X : (these are the heavy items in your bag and if they are at the top, they might squish your other items or make your bag collapse):

These people should be taken out of your bag and avoided.

Now write those that have a check and also a circle. These should be at the bottom of the bag so it doesn't squish the other items or rot and spread the rot to other items, at least until they can respect your new lifestyle and boundaries:

It's important to have a discussion with these people, clearly identify your boundaries, and ask they don't use around you or offer any substance to you.

If they can respect that, perfect. If they can't, they need to be out of your bag of influence and stay away from them until they can respect your boundaries and new lifestyle.

CHAPTER 16: CHALLENGING YOUR THOUGHTS

Changing your approach to negative thoughts that keep you stuck.

We often have thoughts and then decide to interpret them without facts. This is dangerous, and it can send us down a rabbit hole of negative thoughts. Have you ever had a situation where you text someone, and they didn't reply right away, your mind automatically went to,

"They don't like me, and they are ignoring me, they don't appreciate me. What did I do to them??"

Then a few hours later, they message you saying, "sorry, I just saw your message I was at the hospital."

Or, "just saw your message I was in meetings all day or with a sick child."

Or how often have you convinced yourself to do something then regretted it? In the moment, those thoughts seemed like facts, but afterward, you see the other options and that it wasn't a fact it was an unconscious choice or interpretation.

Challenging your thoughts is a key part in reprogramming your brain that will allow you to change your perspective on life and issues that arise. This will help you slowly start shifting your automatic mindset from negative thoughts, perceptions, and interpretations to a more positive outlook, perception, and interpretations. With time positive will become the new normal and life will be brighter and more beautiful.

Challenging your thoughts is very important with the whole family and loved ones. When we have a loved one in active addiction, we often become discouraged or hopeless, and our mind frame shifts from hope to hopeless. This often causes us to start interpreting situations in a more negative manner.

For example, we are used to sitting by the phone waiting for a call from the person going through the addiction to know they are ok, or for the cops to call saying they are not ok. And so we make up these scenarios in our mind as to why they haven't called. This causes a lot of anxiety and frustration in the family system.

So, once our loved one is out of active addiction and starts the journey to a healthy recovery lifestyle, we have to start challenging our thoughts. We need to reprogram to avoid going on autopilot and automatically drawing negative interpretations of a situation or issue.

Yes, in the past, when our loved one was in the active addiction maybe something could have happened to them. But either way these are all things we have no control over and making scenarios up causes extra grief and anxiety. Now that our loved one is on the path of recovery we must get on that path also and start recognizing how we have no control over other people and only over our actions. Challenging our thoughts will allow us to regain our positive outlook on life and our trust in our love done.

CHAPTER 17: BREAKING THE CYCLE OF ADDICTION

Tearing down patterns that keep you in active addiction.

The Cycle of Addiction Exercise

If a situation arises and you get upset or triggered. Fill in the below chart to help figure out thoughts and facts.

What is the situation?

- Trigger: What happened?
- Feeling: What emotion did I feel?
- Body: Where did I feel it in my body? What did it feel like?
- Thoughts: What were my thoughts? What stories did I fabricate?
- Actions: What did I do? What actions did I take?
- Gain: What did I gain from those actions?
- Cost: What did this decision cost me?

Determine how that cost made you feel and go through the list again. Continue to do this over and over until you identify a reason strong enough to step out of this cycle.

By doing this exercise regularly, it will allow you to identify thoughts and facts more naturally and will help you reconnect with your body and emotions so you can step out of the addiction cycle before it begins or shortly after.

**The Cycle of addiction was taught to me by Valerie Mason John in her MBAR program (Mindfulness Based Addiction Recovery) it was very helpful in my recovery, and I've used a modified version of it with clients since.

CHAPTER 18: EXERCISE

**Creating an exercise routine
that will support your recovery.**

Exercise and physical activity are a critical part of a healthy and effective recovery lifestyle. At this point, it's important to introduce a minimum of 30 minutes of exercise or physical activity per day into your daily routine.

Exercise can be done at home or a gym in solo or a group fitness or boot camp groups.

Physical activity can be a sport, running, walking, hiking, yoga, or physical labor. Any activity that allows you to sweat and get your dopamine flowing.

Why is this so important? In active addiction we often use substances that will trick our brain into releasing more dopamine or serotonin. When we start our recovery lifestyle journey it's important to find other ways to get our Dopamine firing. Physical activity is a great way to achieve that, and it's great for our mind and body. If we lack dopamine, it can be dangerous for relapse, so why not prevent it by including physical activity in our daily routine. I often recommend to client if they have a craving to stop and do 20 squats, pushups or jumping jacks. This will give a quick rush of dopamine that can allow you the clear mind needed to make a good choice regarding using.

As for family and loved ones, introducing physical activity will be great to model the action, but also it will allow you to fill in some down times with physical activity that will help you feel better inside and out and give you more energy to tackle life.

What does integrating physical activity and exercise every day look like for you?

When in your weekly plan will you introduce exercise and physical activity?

Exercise plan courtesy André Daigle, Peak Fitness.

Head on over to www.TheRecoveryLifestyle.ca and join our Book Club! You'll receive a detailed Functional Movement Exercise Plan designed to support your recovery success!

CHAPTER 19:
SELF-CARE

**Learning to love, respect,
and care for yourself first.**

It is important to do self-care regularly. In recovery we need to learn to love ourselves, respect ourselves and care for us first before others.

This is important for the person going through the addiction because, in active addiction, we tend to forget how important caring for ourselves is. We forget how great it feels to give ourselves love since we have been seeking love and comfort from outside sources for so long.

Our time and energy are spent finding, hiding, and using our substance of choice. We come to a point where we don't care about ourselves and often distract ourselves from our feelings and thoughts by helping others or using to get temporary relief from being with ourselves.

By introducing self-care as part of our daily routine, it allows our brain to start experiencing good feelings and rewards without the use of a substance. This can help the programming process of your pleasure center.

This is also very important for the family and loved ones of the person going through addiction. It allows you to model self-care to the person going through addiction. And it goes with the saying, but actions speak louder than words.

It's also important to introduce self-care in our daily lives since often we end up forgetting about ourselves, our needs and taking time for self-care since we are so busy worrying and caring for our loved one that is going through addiction. So now that we no longer need to worry and care for that person, it's a good idea to fill that time with self-care and hobbies to prevent our family system from relapsing into enabling and codependent behaviors.

What is self-care, in your opinion? (Write your definition here.)

A simple way to define self-care:

Self-care is mindfully or consciously taking your time and energy to take care of you, to love and tend to you. Not in a selfish way, in a self-love kind of way. Like we would take time every day to care and tend to our child or loved ones, but instead, we take that time to focus on ourselves and honor ourselves by caring for ourselves.

In your opinion, is self-care selfish or self-centered?

It might feel selfish or self-centered to start, but it is not, it is part of being healthy and having boundaries. We can't pour from an empty glass, so we need to care for ourselves to ensure our glass is always full before we help others.

List ten things that come to mind that you could incorporate into your life to practice self-care:

1.

2.

3.

4.

5.

6.

7.

8.

9.

10.

Now circle your top five self-care activities that feel the most exciting or beneficial to you.

How will you incorporate these into your new lifestyle?

How often should you practice self-care?

Incorporate a minimum of 30 minutes per day of self-care. This is 30 minutes you block off in your day just for you, a date with yourself.

Self-care is also setting personal boundaries for ourselves and others around us out of love and respect for ourselves.

List five non-negotiable boundaries you think are important in your life and for your health and welfare, then enforce them and respect them and make sure you communicate your boundaries to your loved ones so they can also respect your boundaries.

1.

2.

3.

4.

5.

CHAPTER 20: BUDGETING

Creating a financial plan to stand on your own two feet.

In active addiction, we often only have one focus, and it's to find money so we can use. Budgeting is not a priority. But once we stop using, we need to learn to budget our money so we can live in society, so we can pay our bills, pay for our necessities and also have some leftover for very important self-care.

Depending on your knowledge and comfort zone on budgeting and personal finance, it's important to remember it's ok to ask for help in this aspect or any aspect of creating your recovery lifestyle.

This aspect is very important since often in active addiction, we become very good at finding ways to make money, but we never learn to save up because we have become wired for instant gratification.

Same goes for family members and loved ones. Often, we are good at managing our finances except when it comes to giving money to the person going through addiction because often we feel we can't say no. That usually leads to us as a family system incorporating an amount in our budget to help the person going through the addiction.

This exercise can help take back control of your money and allocate those funds to another part of your life like your self-care.

If you are the one going thru the addiction, this will help you have a birds-eye view of your financial situation and where you are spending your money so you can make life changes needed to help with your new Recovery Lifestyle and help you attain your goals.

Below is a budgeting template you can use to get an overview of your finances, see where or if the budget is out of balance and make adjustments, and find solutions. You can use this template, create your own or use some budgeting software that you can find online, such as, Mint.com or youneedabudget.com

> *Head on over to www.TheRecoveryLifestyle.ca and join our Book Club! You'll receive a free Budget Template from Liette Collier of Seize the Day Life Coaching!*

CHAPTER 21:
RELAPSE PREVENTION

Protecting the investment
of your recovery lifestyle.

Now that you have created a strong recovery lifestyle and routine, you will want to protect the investment of time and money you have put into your recovery.

Relapse prevention is also important for the family and loved ones of a person going through addiction. The person going through the addiction will work at preventing relapse to the substance or behavior or emotional relapse. The family and loved ones will work at preventing relapse, enabling behaviors and codependency to help foster a family dynamic that is conducive to recovery for everyone.

I've seen too many times clients that work hard on their recovery only to go back to a family system that is not well, where no other loved ones got on the recovery lifestyle journey. This situation often makes it very difficult for the person going through the addiction to stay on the path of recovery.

If the whole family and loved ones embark on the journey together, it makes it easier for everyone and allows more open discussion and more understanding. If the family and loved ones don't embark on the journey and expect the person going through the addiction to do it alone, this often leads to adding more pressure and unrealistic expectations put on the one going through the addiction. Often, the loved one that was most codependent on the one going through the addiction ends up unconsciously jeopardizing the person's recovery to fulfill their self-worth issues. With that said, sometimes we have no control over who our loved ones are and their actions. If you are the one going through the addiction and your loved ones don't want to be part of the recovery process, it's ok as long as you build a good support network.

I've also seen many clients in this situation and although it can be frustrating, stay positive. Keep focusing on yourself and things you have control over and set good boundaries to prevent your loved ones from affecting your recovery.

Sometimes that means taking your distance from certain loved ones. This can be short term and sometimes long term. But in the end, it's important to do everything in your power and control for your recovery.

You have control over the decisions and choices you make regarding your health and recovery lifestyle, so make sure to make informed decisions, not emotional decisions.

Key things to remember in relapse preventions:

- Vulnerability is a strength. Ask for help.

- You have the power to decide if you want to use or not.

- Use your tools.

- Have a list of emergency contacts.

- Have your list of guiding principles.

- Honor yourself by sitting with the uncomfortable feeling or craving and know it's not permanent. It will pass.

- Have a list of activities you can do to help get your mind off things, regulate your emotions and stop stinking thinking.

- If you pick up, know you have the option at any time to put it back down and use the relapse, lapse or slip as a learning experience.

List 7 activities you can do to get your mind calmed temporarily if emotions or cravings get too intense:

1.

2.

3.

4.

5.

6.

7.

Make a list of 3 positive influencers you can contact if you are in crisis, danger of picking-up, triggered or emotional crisis:

1.

2.

3.

Make a list of signs and trigger behaviors that indicates you are at risk of relapse, triggered or emotionally struggling. Then share this with the people closest to you so they can help you recognize the signs.

1.

2.

3.

4.

5.

6.

7.

Triggers can be many things like sounds, taste, smells, people, situations, things, places, or even lack of sleep.

Signs of being triggered can vary from person to person but can be things like a change in sleeping patterns or eating patterns, change in attitude, emotionally unstable, pushing friends away, loss of interests you like, isolating or even surplus of energy or romanticizing about your substance of choice.

CHAPTER 22:
JOURNALING

Using journaling to build self-awareness and to limit negative thinking.

Journaling is a good tool to help you be more self-aware and keep track of how your feeling and if your progress. Journaling is also beneficial because it allows you to put what's going on in your mind all that stinking thinking out on paper so you can focus on the positive and reach your goals. It can also be a great way to uncover patterns that might be detrimental to your recovery.

Journaling should be done daily, even if it's just writing one sentence that includes how your day was, any events that happened, if you feel good, bad, or neutral about the events and your overall emotional state. This is just a guideline. You can write whatever you feel like writing in journal.

I've seen many clients that are struggling with addiction as well as families of clients struggling with addiction suffer from anxiety or having a difficult time falling asleep because of the stinking thinking stuck in a vicious cycle in their head.

After implementing a daily journaling practice, they reported having a significant improvement in their sleep and anxiety just by taking the thoughts out of their head and putting them on paper.

It's also a great resource to help find patterns or to help remind you of things you might forget to mention when meeting with a therapist or recovery coach.

When thoughts wander in our minds, it's sometimes easy for us to convince ourselves of what we want, good or bad, simply to shut those thoughts off.

When we put it on paper, it helps to make it real and allows us to deal with it more subjectively and not just push it away temporarily like we would if we let the thought cycle in our mind.

CHAPTER 23: FINDING HOBBIES

Create 'feel good' moments in your week that will support recovery.

It's very important to incorporate hobbies in our weekly schedule as soon as possible when setting up our Recovery Lifestyle.

This will allow us to create new connections, feel positive and experience happy moments that can help change our perspective on life.

I had a client who said he didn't have any passions or hobbies he liked. This was one of the reasons why he felt depressed and anxious. Every day he woke up with no plans and nothing to look forward to. Trying to stay sober was proving to be difficult because he was staying in his room and had nothing to do but to be with his thoughts. Thoughts that over the years had been trained to think of using and finding his substance of choice.

Every day he felt overwhelmed. He had nothing in his life that brought him joy and got his mind doing something else than ruminating over drugs. But then we went through the exercises on the following pages to help find that spark and that passion. The moment he remembered he enjoyed the gym and how going to the gym use to make him feel was amazing to witness. His eyes lit up talking about it. So he integrated going to the gym in his weekly schedule, and within a week he could feel the difference, and I could see a difference in his posture and mind frame.

That opened up the door to remembering other activities he enjoyed and the skills he has like online investing. This allowed us to create an action plan to achieve the goal of having enough funds to start investing online again. This example is meant to show you that shining light on one passion or hobby can start the ball rolling for many other great "Aha" moments that help strengthen our recovery.

Why is finding hobbies so important?

- A great way to fill spare time in a healthy and constructive way. When we start a new Recovery Lifestyle, we often end up having a lot of spare time on our hands since we cut out people, places, things, and activities that were not healthy or conducive to our new Recovery lifestyle, values, and life goals.

- Are a great way to meet like-minded people outside of recovery groups and build new healthy connection.

- Can help us feel a sense of self-worth and of belonging to something.

- Can be a healthy coping mechanism to help us through hard times or emotions.

- Can be a great stress relief a great way to temporarily get away from life stressors.

- It can challenge your limits and provide you with small wins that help us feel good.

Write a list of seven hobbies you'd like to try.

If you're having a hard time thinking of ideas, visit Wikipedia, and search "List of Hobbies."

1.

2.

3.

4.

5.

6.

7.

CHAPTER 24:
ACTION PLANNING

Creating a definitive plan to
regain control of your life.

The Action Plan is as important for the loved ones as it is for the person going through the addiction.

As a loved one, your action plan will help you regain your life. It will help prevent codependency and enabling behaviors since everyone will be focusing on their self-care, life, and finding there happy lifestyle that suits them.

The action plan gives everyone involved in the recovery process direction so everyone can work together to achieve their personal goals.

It helps model the work needed to achieve a healthy recovery lifestyle to other members of the family, including the one going through the addiction.

Also having an Action plan can help relieve some anxiety associated with not knowing what direction we are going with our life. This helps us make our daily decisions more effectively because we will have our action plan in mind.

Why is having goals and an action plan important?

- A goal without an action plan is called a dream, and it remains a dream until a plan of action is made to make that dream become a reality.

- Having goals helps to give our lives purpose and meaning.

- Waking up with purpose and hope gives us energy and joy for our day.

- Having a goal and action plan allows us to work towards making better decisions in our day to day life. We can evaluate our decisions based on if it will bring us closer to our goals or push us away from our goals. After all, our life journey is woven together with every decision we make.

- Having an action plan and goals allows us to achieve our goals and celebrate the accomplishment. This helps us feel good, boosts our self-esteem and self-love.

- Having NO plan and NO goals are the biggest mistakes some will make in their recovery lifestyle. This can quickly lead to relapse or bad choices that go against our values and core principles. So, dream, set a plan, and transform those dreams into reality.

The Action Plan is as important for the loved ones as it is for the person going through the addiction.

As a loved one, your action plan will help you regain your life. It will help prevent codependency and enabling behaviors since everyone will be focusing on their self-care, life and finding there happy lifestyle that suits them.

NEXT STEPS

Congratulations on taking the big step to recover your life.

The first big decision is the one you made when you picked up this book. Now you are on the right path to live the life you desire, the life you deserve.

I encourage you to follow the steps, strategies, and exercises I have outlined in this book. They can help you build a solid recovery foundation, helping you to find success, however you define success.

I invite you to connect with me directly. I especially want to hear your stories of success, and your stories of challenge. I'm here to tell you, you are not in this alone.

I also would love to hear your feedback about the book and the exercises outlined within, I am always looking to improve them. I want to know what works, and what doesn't work for you.

And finally, please go to my website, www.TheRecoveryLifestyle.ca. There you will find downloads mentioned in the book, special worksheets, and more... all free.

Sign up for our "Book Club" and you'll receive budget templates, additional exercises, meal plans, and bonus materials we just couldn't include in the book. And, we are always coming up with new ways to support you on your recovery journey.

Join

THE RECOVERY
LIFESTYLE

Book Club

Book Updates, Worksheets,
Meal Plans, Bonus Exercises...
All Free!

www.TheRecoveryLifestyle.ca

ACKNOWLEDGEMENTS

I would like to thank:

My parents, brother, and sister for always believing in me and never giving up.

The team at Trafalgar Residence for their help and guidance when I was at my most vulnerable state. Especially Sydney Bater and Souha Bawab, the two most amazing, compassionate, and talented psychotherapists. I was truly blessed to have you guide me on my journey to healing.

Laura Crawford, for helping me heal my insides while educating me and helping me grow spiritually and to believe in myself.

Dr. Cali Estes for sharing her knowledge and passion with me and be a great role model and mentor.

Dr. Valerie Mason-John for being a great inspiration, mentor, and friend.

Stephanie Sutherland for helping me and guiding me to make this dream of writing a book a reality.

James Hamilton Healy and his publishing company for making this journey so easy and stress free.

An anonymous family friend that saved my life by advancing me the money so I could go to a private rehab.

And a big thank you to all the sponsors that helped me fund this book anonymously out of the grace of their hearts to do their part in helping those struggling and their families.

ABOUT THE AUTHOR

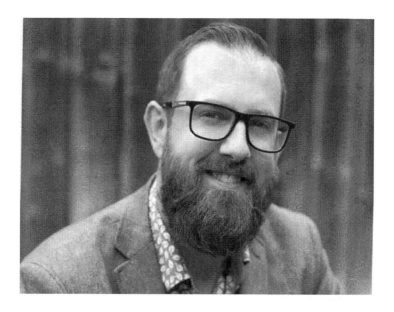

Mr. André Viel is a certified Recovery Coach, Family Recovery Coach, and Interventionist. His business, Hope Recovery Coaching, is striving to be one of the programs that can help those suffering from substance use disorder and other mental health issues find the path they need to do just that, heal and stop.

More information:

www.TheRecoveryLifestyle.ca

www.NeverGiveUpHope.ca